PLANT BASED DIET FOR BEGINNERS

The Beginner's Guild Book on How to Prepare Delicious and Consume Your Healthy Meal to Help Lose Weight and Live Your Best

JAMES ARNOLD

Table of Contents

CHAPTER ONE

INTRODUCTION

Are you curious about what precisely a plant-based diet is, how to get began, and a way to make it stick? If so, you've come to the proper location. I've created this reachable plant-based eating regimen newbie's guide, so you will have all the information you need, right at your fingertips.

Ingesting a plant-based weight loss plan means getting maximum or all of your energy from sparkling, whole plant meals that are minimally processed (or maybe better, no longer processed in any respect). Basically, it's miles exactly what it sounds like — a eating regimen made from normally vegetation.

A plant-primarily based weight loss plan also can be vegetarian or vegan, but these diets aren't necessarily outright plant-based totally. There are masses of "junk food vegans" who may not consume animal merchandise, but still eat an expansion of processed meals.

CHAPTER TWO

WHAT TO CONSUME ON A PLANT-BASED DIET

When picturing what a plant-based meal looks like, fruits and greens possibly come to thoughts. And that they're a critical part of pretty much any healthy food regimen. But you're no longer constrained to these ingredients. There are extensive kinds of plant meals to enjoy.

The major sorts of meals usually eaten on a plant-based food plan include:

- End result — Ex: Apples, berries, kiwis, mangoes, avocado, bananas, jackfruit, and so forth.

- Greens — Ex: Onions, broccoli, beets, potatoes, mushrooms, carrots, and so forth.

- Whole grains — Ex: Quinoa, millet, buckwheat, wheat, rice, corn, etc.

- Beans & legumes — Ex: Black beans, chickpeas, lentils, edamame, peas, and so forth.

- Nuts & seeds — Ex: Almonds, cashews, chia seeds, flaxseeds, walnuts, and many others.

- Herbs & spices – Ex: Turmeric, ginger, cinnamon, oregano, garlic, cayenne, and so on.

- Fermented meals – Ex: Kimchi, sauerkraut, miso, natto, etc.

Eating throughout a majority of these meals agencies will assist you get an abundance of micronutrients out of your food. Also, when selecting from each category, assume "consume the rainbow." colorful plant ingredients are full of phytochemicals (a fancy word that just means "chemicals from vegetation) and antioxidants which might be right for maintaining unique components of your body healthy.

CHAPTER THREE

WHAT TO AVOID ON A PLANT-BASED DIET

While choosing to consume a plant-based weight loss program, you'll want to focus mainly on sparkling ingredients. In a grocery save, which means normally purchasing the outer aisles. If feasible, choose natural meals as a great deal as feasible to avoid publicity to GMOs and pesticides.

However, the primary ingredients you must keep away from on a plant-primarily based diet are:

•	Most or all animal merchandise (particularly manufacturing unit-farmed meat, eggs, & dairy merchandise)

•	Refined sugars (White sugar, cane sugar, excessive fructose corn syrup, chemical-based totally calorie-loose sweeteners, etc.)

•	pretty processed vegetable oils (Corn oil, cottonseed oil, sunflower oil, peanut oil, soybean oil, and many others.)

•	White flour (particularly bleached white flour which is full of chemical compounds and heavy metals — and genuinely without nutrients)

•   Junk food (which includes maximum cookies, chips, crackers, snack bars, sweetened beverages, packaged meals, and so on.)

•   GMOs   (The   primary genetically engineered plants are corn, soy, canola, sugar beets, cotton, and alfalfa — plus a piece of apple, zucchini, and potato)

You'll also need to pay special interest to nutrients labels. By means of studying labels, you could keep away from ultra-processed   and   dangerous components. Packaged foods need to have as few components as viable. As a preferred rule, if you can't pronounce an element, or don't realize what it's far, put the food back.

CHAPTER FOUR

GLUTEN & GRAINS

For most of the people, grains can be part of a healthy, plant-based food plan. Some of my favorites are quinoa, millet, amaranth, buckwheat, oats, and teff. In lots of studies, complete grains were shown to help fight coronary heart sickness, type 2 diabetes, most cancers, and even obesity. But now not everything is peachy in grain land.

Maximum of the grains eaten inside the global nowadays are

sprayed with pesticides, and some plants, specifically wheat, can also even be handled with glyphosate as a desiccant (to dry the crop out before harvest). Corn, until it's grown organically, is often genetically engineered. Then there's rice, which, even as popular, is regularly infected with a worrying amount of arsenic.

For a few scientific situations, like autoimmune sicknesses, grains can also reason infection inside the gut and contribute to signs. That is specifically genuine with the gluten found in wheat. despite the fact that handiest about 1% of the sector's populace has recognized celiac sickness, many more show signs and symptoms of gluten intolerance with signs like complications, joint ache, skin issues, seizures, and digestive problems. In case you're dealing with any of those signs and symptoms, it is able to be helpful to head gluten-free for 3 to six months and see in the event that they resolve.

At the same time as many human beings have jumped at the gluten-free bandwagon, that doesn't mean it's always best for all of us. A few researches genuinely show fitness benefits from consuming whole grain wheat products.

in case you're going to eat wheat, although, you may want to search for 100% whole wheat (on account that white flour doesn't do your frame any favors!), and aim to make sure your grains are organically grown, so that you can keep away from glyphosate contamination.

As you begin your adventure on a plant-based eating regimen, you may start to get questions from buddies and circle of relatives. Any time you devour in a different way than the norm, you're sure to get some pushback.

It's like, you may consume fast meals for every meal for 10 years and no one will bat an eye fixed. But change a fried hen meal for a inexperienced salad topped with sunflower seeds, and anybody abruptly issues approximately you shriveling up and wasting away.

Many people agree with you may not get all the vitamins you need without animal merchandise. But plant life has protein, calcium, and iron in abundance, further to a number of different nutrients, minerals, and antioxidants. (And sure, many flowers are considerable sources of choline.) In actuality, people nowadays are a ways more likely to be poor in fiber than protein: simplest 3% of American citizens get their every day quantity of recommended fiber. However that's no longer a problem when you're eating primarily flowers!

Dietary supplements

No matter how you pick out to consume, inside the modern global, most diets are lacking in something. In the case of plant-primarily based diets, there are a few nutrients which might be in particular crucial to pay attention to.

They're:

- Nutrition B12

- Diet D3

- Omega-three fatty acids

- Nutrition K2

- Zinc

Inside the case of those vitamins, supplements can be necessary to keep away from a deficiency.

CHAPTER FIVE

HEALTH ADVANTAGES OF PLANT-BASED DIET

Consuming the right ingredients and getting the vitamins your frame desires is essential to proper health. And adopting a plant-primarily based weight-reduction plan will positioned you on the short tune to fitness and power.

Costs of chronic ailment are accelerating at an alarming fee. And it's taking place in human beings more youthful and more youthful. Unfortunately, in step with the sector fitness organization (WHO), with the aid of 2020, chronic illnesses will account for nearly 3-quarters of all deaths worldwide. This consists of diseases like most cancers, coronary heart sickness, type 2 diabetes, Alzheimer's, autoimmune disease, and digestive disorders, amongst many others.

But thanks to the studies of plant-powered Adopting a plant-based diet advantages many elements of fitness, including the subsequent:

Coronary heart ailment

Following a plant-based totally food plan has been shown to undoubtedly advantage those with cardiovascular ailment. Research, that found that the greater plant protein, legumes, and veggies humans ate, the less possibly they were to die of coronary artery disease.

Through eating more end result and veggies and less meat (especially beef) you may save you damage to the cells that line and protect your blood vessels. Within the previous few decades, science has determined that damage to this endothelial lining causes specific styles of heart sickness and atherosclerosis.

Type 2 Diabetes

Changing animal protein with plant protein has a profound high quality effect on humans with type 2 diabetes. Whilst researchers reviewed and analyzed the records from thirteen randomized managed trials, they located a decrease in three crucial markers of diabetic severity — hemoglobin A1C, fasting glucose, and fasting insulin — whilst switching from animal protein to plant protein.

A observe on the results of a low-fats vegan weight loss program on people dwelling with type 2 diabetes. He showed that eating this way improved weight loss, blood sugar manage, and triglyceride ranges in comparison to the eating regimen advocated by using the yank Diabetic association.

Even as many humans mistakenly believe that diabetes is as a result of sugar on my own, we are coming to apprehend the position saturated fat performs in its improvement. When type 2 diabetics stop consuming meat (a prime contributing source of saturated fats), their blood sugar tiers generally improve.

Alzheimer's & Neurodegenerative ailment

Accept as true with it or not, even Alzheimer's and neurodegenerative disorder patients can gain from a plant-primarily based eating regimen. At the same time as there are few documented cases of reversal, most are preventable. In fact, over

90% of Alzheimer's instances are preventable.

Tons of this prevention is viable with lifestyle strategies, and entire ingredients plant-primarily based vitamins is one of the most consequential strategies of all. Extra research has proven that this could be due in component to the mind-gut connection. A poor diet disrupts the gut microbiota, contributing to infection inside the body and affecting the important worried gadget and, in the end, the mind. One examine located that irritation, gut dysbiosis, and leaky intestine may contribute to the procedure of neurodegeneration in Alzheimer's patients.

CHAPTER SIX

PREVENTING CANCER WITH PLANT-BASED DIET

Plant-primarily based diets can help prevent cancer too. A 2011 study concluded that a plant-based diet (which includes vegan and vegetarian ones) are a beneficial method to reduce your threat of cancer. Particularly, the increased intakes of plant life, removal of crimson and processed meats, and maintenance of a healthy body have been attributed to a reduction in most cancers.

Some plant foods that show in particular strong anticancer outcomes are:

Nuts

A chief look at showed that individuals who ate nuts extensively decreased their chance of most cancers (and normal mortality) compared to folks that ate few or no nuts. Additionally, the yank Society of medical Oncology released a report of more than 800 sufferers with level III colon most cancers. They observed that eating nuts can make a giant difference in basic most cancers survival. in the have a look at, people who fed on approximately 2 small handfuls (approximately 2 ounces) of tree nuts in keeping with week had a forty six% lower danger of cancer recurrence and a 53% decrease hazard of demise than people who did not devour nuts.

Cooked Tomatoes

The cancer-combating energy of tomatoes may be resulting from lycopene, a most cancers-starving antioxidant. Studies show that guys who eat 2 to 3 cups of cooked tomatoes twice weekly have a 30% diminished threat of prostate cancer.

Purple Potatoes

once a food of the Incan kings, red potatoes include a natural chemical called anthocyanin, which starves and kills cancer cells — and wipes out the scary cancer stem cells.

Mushrooms

Researchers from the University of Western Australia in Perth performed a take a look at of 2,000 Chinese ladies. (About half of had suffered from breast most cancers.) The scientists reviewed the ladies' ingesting conduct and factored out other variables that make a contribution to most cancers, inclusive of being obese, lack of exercise, and smoking. They came to a startling finding approximately mushrooms. girls who fed on at the least a 3rd of an oz. of clean mushrooms every day (approximately one mushroom consistent with day) were 64% less likely to increase breast most cancers. While the ones equal women additionally drank green tea day by day, they reduced their threat of breast most cancers by 89%.

Weight problems

Quotes of weight problems are at an all-time excessive round the world. Inside the U.S. on my own, over 39% of the population is affected by weight problems. Ingesting a plant-based diet enables fight weight problems, too.

A 16-week randomized clinical trial showed that a plant-based vegan food regimen contributes to a discount in frame weight, fats mass, and insulin resistance. And a observe posted inside the British journal of nutrients concluded that each extra yr of adopting a vegan food regimen reduced the chance of obesity by 7%. That's nothing to sneeze at.

CHAPTER SEVEN

PLANT-BASED TOTALLY EATING REGIMEN BENEFITS TO THE SURROUNDINGS

Adopting a plant-based totally weight loss plan isn't just excellent on your fitness; it's additionally true for our planet. Cycling energy through livestock is a lot much less efficient than consuming them directly. It takes about 12 kilos of grain or soy to provide one pound of feedlot pork. For beef, it takes about seven pounds of feed to produce one pound of safe to eat meat, and for hen, about four. No marvel 80% of the arena's soy crop and 70% of the grain grown in the U.S. is being fed to feed cattle.

Animal agriculture is, basically, a protein manufacturing facility in reverse.

Worldwide, about 8 times as a lot land is used to grow food for animals as is used to grow food for human beings. Huge tracts of forest are being cut down to make manner for manufacturing unit farms, areas for cows to graze, or fields to grow animal feed.

If the world, simply hypothetically, went vegan, we'd loose up 75% of the globe's agricultural land — a place the dimensions of the Us, Australia, the ecu Union, China, and India blended. That land may be used to grow meals for a unexpectedly expanding human populace, can be planted with timber or other plant life to soak up carbon out of the environment, can be back to natural world, or may be used for lots other functions.

Current practices in animal agriculture contribute substantially to global greenhouse fuel emissions, too. And while CO2 is one main issue, it isn't the handiest one. As national Geographic places it, methane, the gasoline that comes out of a cow's plumbing, is even extra efficient than CO2 at trapping heat. 28 instances more powerful, to be exact. Not most effective that but in an international facing a probably irreversible weather disaster, methane dissipates a lot greater swiftly than CO2. Meaning changing your weight-reduction plan these days will reduce your carbon footprint right now.

THE END

www.ingramcontent.com/pod-product-compliance
Lightning Source LLC
Chambersburg PA
CBHW051406150726
48000CB00003B/1348